NUTRITION FOR HEALTHY LIFE

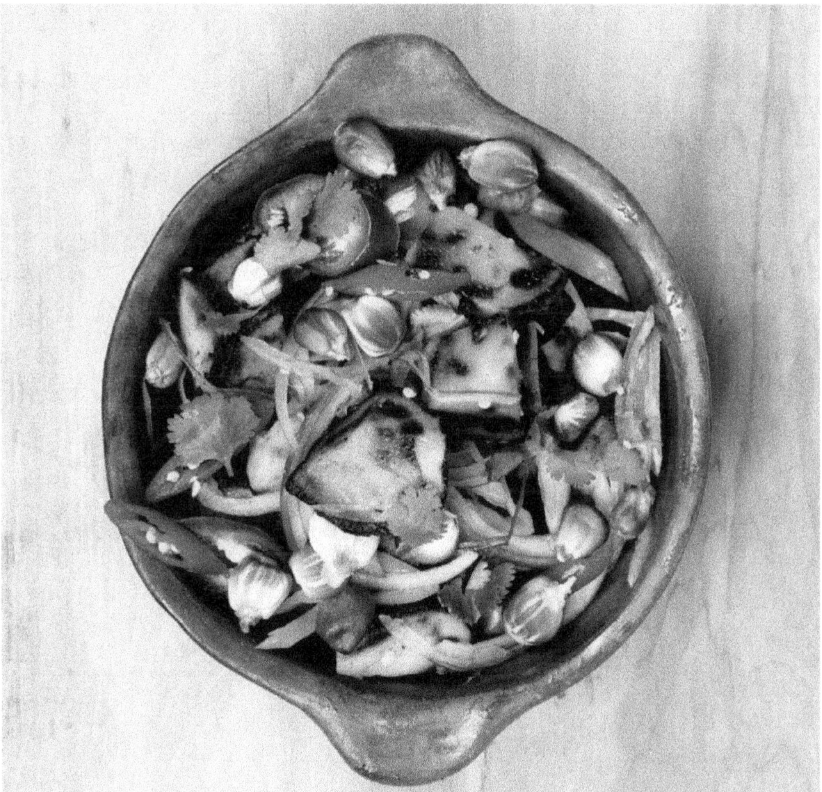

DR. JOHN ADAMS

Contents

INTRODUCTION

Foreword

Simply said, the body's two distinct and intricate processes for generating energy are significantly different from one another. The two-energy style depends on one another for support because energy is essential to human activity and survival. You can learn which foods in this book can provide you the greatest energy.

We often make the decision to start a health and fitness program with enthusiasm and perhaps a lot of hype, but after the first week, everything starts to fizzle out. Why don't we follow through with our diet goals, morning jog programs, and fitness plans that we make?

What can we do, for our own sakes as well as the sakes of others who depend on us, to ensure that we continue with our plans?

Do you eat merely to save your hunger or to please your taste buds? Or do you eat in order to have more control over your life? This eBook demonstrates how focusing on eating properly may greatly improve your quality of life.

CHAPTER 1 THE BAICS

Energy is required for a number of activities like maintaining growth, everyday tasks, exercise, and several other motions or functions that are sometimes taken for granted. Both of the energy systems utilize them.

Rarely do any health and exercise plans in the modern world actually work. What is the cause of their alarmingly high failure rate? Two decades ago, the globe was more healthier than it is today. This is largely related to peoples' changing eating patterns.

The Basics

The aerobic system is the main and first to be used energy system. This system makes a lot of demands on the body as a whole and needs oxygen to power the muscles. Due to the concomitant rise in heart rate, this requirement typically causes an increase in the rate, depth, and blood supply.

The body's system naturally switches to the anaerobic energy system when it needs more energy than it can supply because it demands more oxygen than usual. This device has the ability to generate energy without using oxygen.

All of this energy is produced through appropriate or sensible food consumption. The types of energy levels that each person can produce depend on the foods consumed. When all available energy sources have been used up, muscle weariness usually sets in for a variety of reasons, the most compelling one being the kinds of foods that have been ingested.

It is important to note the foods that develop or boost the energy generating sources because there are many food categories that offer different health benefits for the human body system. The person should be able to select the appropriate foods with the use of this knowledge.

The anaerobic system releases energy from nutrients stored in the body, typically during severe activity bouts, whereas the aerobic system breaks down the curbs, fatty acids, and amino acids in the foods consumed. If we hear about diet or exercise failures all around us, it's usually not their fault.

In many cases, it is the responsibility of the people who made a big deal out of following these programs in the beginning, telling all of their friends and coworkers about it. Naturally, those who drop out of a fitness or diet program midway do not perceive the benefits, and everyone blames the program.

Not a brand-new diet or exercise regimen, but motivation is what the world needs right now. To carry out whatever strategy they have chosen all the way through, the right mindset is required.

If they can accomplish that, the majority of health problems linked to lifestyle choices will become obsolete. The best part is that we don't need to travel far to find this drive. We just need to look inside and use the motivation that is already inside of us.

People wouldn't have dreamed of buying whatever junk food they could acquire to feed their faces a generation ago. Today, we act in that manner extremely casually. When someone says, "I'm hungry," they typically mean, "I want a burger or a hot dog, perhaps with chips and some coke." Furthermore, saying "I'm on a diet" actually means "I'm taking a chemical-laden tablet that will snuff out my hunger and deprive my body of vitamins." There is really no explanation for why we are currently dealing with so many health difficulties.

Our health is a reflection of the foods we eat. The terrible state in which we find ourselves is a global matter, not just a personal one.

Everyone in the world eats improperly. By the year 2021, eight out of ten people in the US will be overweight, up from the current figure of six out of ten.

Are we really considering this? We're not. You probably have a bag of chips by your side as you read this eBook. Do you realize that the money you spent on that package, which contains some of the most dangerous substances known to man, might have instead been used to feed a malnourished child in Ruanda?

But it goes beyond simply being charitable. It also pertains to us. Yes, we must be self-centered. Are we on the verge of a catastrophe with such horrifying health statistics? We definitely aren't eating properly. We must be ready for any excess baggage that comes with obesity and the various illnesses it leaves behind.

So keep this in mind the next time you see software failing or drawing a lot of negative attention: it's not likely that the program is unstable. Most of the time, it was a result of people starting out with good intentions but not finishing the program as they should have.

CHAPTER

2THE WAY YOU THINK ABOUT FOOD

Even more important than a trainer or a doctor, your personal motivation is what you need to keep your health and fitness program going. To carefully examine the situation, you must be committed. You are therefore looking to lose a few pounds because you are overweight.

If you don't take the necessary steps to have the proper diet and to adhere to your regular exercise schedule, no gym instructor from anywhere in the world will be able to help you. No doctor will be able to help you, even if you are unwell and seeking treatment, if you are not committed to adhering to the recommended course of action, whether that involves taking medication at the recommended time or avoiding certain foods.

Your Mentality

So far, we have deviated drastically from our normal dietary patterns. Things won't go better unless we assess the situation and take action on our own.

The most important factor is awareness. We must educate ourselves about which foods are healthy for us and which are not. We need to go back to our training to understand what nutrients, and in what quantities, your body actually needs.

Then, in order to create a diet plan for ourselves and our loved ones that would allow us to eat healthily, We need to eat fewer foods that are bad for us—sugars, fats, and carbohydrates are things we don't really need—and more foods that could improve our health.

I realize that this does sound a bit overly preachy. However, that is the only break we have. We'll never get better as long as we keep eating Oreos. Still, there is hope.

There are many things that are just as tasty as those dreadful junk foods, but we are just learning about them, so there is yet hope.

These are the foods we don't yet know about, we probably don't like them, or we don't know how to prepare them, but a healthy cookbook may allow you to understand several intriguing ways to cook healthily. You can create some pretty tasty healthy recipes even with the same type of diet you now follow. All of that is definitely feasible. You can significantly alter your eating patterns while also paying attention to your palate.

The truth is that the weight loss industry has significantly contributed to the decline of the advanced human race. Atkins, Jenny Craig, Zone, and Midi-fast must continue to be sold, thus the media never informs you of how you can take matters into your own hands.

They flashy before-and-after photos of a man with a foot-long sub and then the same man with six pack abs, and they claim that the diet allowed for that. The truth is that we could very easily achieve that as well, without having to spend thousands of dollars on such diets, if we were to get our act together. What must we do, then?

2 general things: - Regulate our intake. Engage in some physical activity.

Is it a difficult task to complete now? Don't we owe that to our body, which has been so helpful to us for so long? Don't we owe it to our loved ones and to ourselves?

CHAPTER 3 HONEY AND WHOLE GRAINS

Honey has been shown to be the energy circle's sole sustaining force over time. It continues to be unparalleled in its ability to produce energy while also benefiting the human body in other ways. The most natural source of energy is honey. In addition to acting as a powerful immune system booster, it also functions as a natural cure for a wide range of diseases.

The natural flow of a human being's daily life cycle depends heavily on energy. Finding reliable and nutritious energy sources is crucial for maintaining your health and happiness.

A Good Pair

Honey's inherent advantages have long been understood and respected. A natural source of carbohydrates, which are an energy source for enhancing performance, endurance, and lowering levels of muscular tiredness, honey also has a nice taste.

For athletes, this is very helpful. The honey's sugar content aids in avoiding weariness both during physical activity and throughout sports enthusiasts' training sessions. Glucose and fructose, which make up these sugars, have separate but complementary roles.

The honey's glucose component often absorbs more quickly and provides an immediate energy boost, whilst the fructose works more slowly and provides a longer-lasting and more sustained energy release. Honey has been shown to assist maintain steady blood sugar levels in the body when it comes to this issue.

Consuming honey is not a particularly tough activity because it is a tasty food item and is natural in its form. In general, people of all ages are eager to consume honey in any of its auxiliary forms. Even little youngsters like it.

A modest amount of honey consumed each day gives kids the energy they need to handle the physical demands of their everyday activities at school and in sports.

Even for adults, ingesting a tiny amount of honey everyday can help maintain optimal energy levels throughout a tough workday. Making honey sandwiches with additional ingredients is one method for coming up with a tasty snack.

Another delicious breakfast option is to spread honey on a slice of freshly baked bread. It is recommended to use honey in place of sugar while making beverages. The majority of people in today's society seek quick fixes for their energy-boosting requirements, which typically come in the form of unhealthy sports drinks, coffee, and processed curbs like sugar and white bread.

Although these give the required boost in energy, it should be noted that this energy is rather fleeting and the fatigue that follows is typically felt more sharply. As a result, choosing to consume whole grains in some form is not only preferable but also significantly healthy.

Whole grains offer energy that is present in a more complex form and breaks down gradually over time. This then establishes the foundation for maintaining energy levels for longer periods of time.

Whole grains have a variety of healthy components because of their more complex makeup, including fiber and a wealth of phytonutrients, minerals, and vitamins. Any dish's flavor is frequently finished off or improved by the addition of whole grain ingredients. There are many different types of whole grains, including wheat, oat, barley, maize, brown rice, faro, spelt, emmer, einkorn, rye, millet, buckwheat, and many more. These can then be used to create a variety of additional products, including tiff flour, whole wheat flour, whole wheat bread, whole wheat pasta, rolled oats or oat grouts, triticale flour, popcorn, and whole wheat flour.

Consistently eating whole grains can help control weight, lower cholesterol levels defend against several types of cancer, and reduce the risk of heart disease. It is important to distinguish whole grains from their inferior and refined "relative." Even though refined grains offer some advantages, whole grain substitutes are always preferable.

CHAPTER 4 NUTS AND LEAN MEAT

Nuts are a significant source of nutrients for intake by both humans and animals. Given its abundance of essential nutrients, it can be consumed raw, cooked, or as a supplement to already prepared foods. Although a nut is typically thought of as a hard-shelled fruit, the nut family also includes a wide variety of other foods.

Different kinds of meat typically contribute to a diversity of flavors, but the healthiest kind is the one that contains the leanest meat. It is undeniable that meets with a substantial level of fat are a gourmet treat, but it is wise to take the time to learn about the advantages of eating lean meats for health reasons.

Good Proteins And Oils

It is now widely known that nuts significantly aid in keeping many illnesses under control or preventing them altogether.

For instance, nuts have been shown to be able to prevent the development of coronary heart disease, even in people who have a long line of relatives who have the condition.

Consuming nuts like almonds and walnuts has been shown to reduce the body's levels of serum cholesterol. Additionally, diabetics and other people with insulin resistance issues should consume nuts.

Another better option is to satisfy cravings with almonds rather than junk food. Another benefit of choosing nuts as a healthier choice is that they contain vital fatty acids. Another benefit of having nuts on hand as snacks is that they are nutritious and may be eaten in their raw form.

Due to its delayed burn properties, which aid to maintain stable blood sugar levels, almonds are frequently used to balance blood lipids. The almond is a well-liked addition to the monotonous diet of the majority of Mediterranean people because it is rich in a variety of different nutrients.

Another healthy nut is the Brazil nut, which has its own advantages when eaten in moderation. The Brazil nut, which is well-known for having omega 3 fatty acids, is also a strong source of calcium.

Another very well-liked nut that is frequently eaten as a salted snack is the cashew nut. However, as it is already a fairly flavored nut on its own, the food item would be much healthier without the salt. These nuts are processed into oils in several regions of the world.

Since relying just on what the unaided eye can see is insufficient, the selecting procedure should be carried out with some understanding. Round, chuck, sirloin, and tenderloin are examples of lean beef cuts, whereas tenderloin, loin chops, and leg are examples of lean hog or lamb cuts. The breast portion without skin would be the leanest part of the bird.

There are many reasons why people choose to omit meat from their diets, but there is no proof that doing so is either healthy or appropriate for everyone.

However, the choice of meats that would make intake healthy—generally speaking, meats with lower fat contents—is the crucial thing to keep in mind here. White meat has a lot less fat than red meat, despite the fact that it is by no means deficient in fat. Lean meats have a wide-ranging, well-rounded nutritional content.

Protein is a very vital component of the basic structural and functional development of every cell nourishment and production and is generally higher and purer in lean meats.

Essential amino acids, notably sulfur amino acids, are also abundant in lean meats. When compared to digestion rates, animal proteins function more quickly than those found in beans and whole grains.

Iron can also be found in lean meat. Because iron deficiency is gradual, it frequently goes undetected until anemia has set in.

CHAPTER 5 THE BENEFIT

Here is all the encouragement you need to keep eating well. Let's start talking about the topic right away.

Advantages

You Get Healthier

Even if we wrote a whole library of books about the health benefits of eating properly, they wouldn't exactly address what benefits actually exist. The main benefit is that you have more control over your weight.

By eating properly, you also ensure that your metabolic processes, most notably your immune system and gastrointestinal system, continue to run smoothly. Additionally, you are guarded against a variety of chronic illnesses, such as diabetes and cardiovascular conditions including coronary artery disease and high blood pressure.

More Cost Effective

Spend substantially less money when you eat healthfully. You notice a significant decrease in your grocery costs, and if you already have credit card debt, you avoid adding to it. Additionally, you save a ton of money on all the medical costs you would incur if a problem resulting from your eating binges arises.

Less Toxins In Your Body

Nowadays, a lot of meals are poisonous due to the synthetic chemicals they contain. One of the fundamental tenets of eating right is that you shouldn't consume any man-made foods, so when you try to eat properly, you are significantly less likely to introduce these poisons into your body.

In addition, cutting back on vices like smoking and drunkenness will be possible if you eat less. A beer nearly always signifies a night out with the guys. You won't crave the beer as much if you eat less. Similar to this, you won't want to smoke one (or more) cigarettes after every meal as is customary.

More Physical Lifestyle

You'll discover that you can function much more effectively when you eat better. You can live a more productive life by getting more exercise, traveling, playing, and working.

That certainly beats being a slob and spending the entire day on the couch, doesn't it? Additionally, you are able to spend more time with your friends and loved ones, which unquestionably

Good Social Life

Forget about the "fat fetishism," overweight people don't look good. The social stigma surrounding having weight in the incorrect places on the body is very strong. Your extra weight can actually hinder your ability to locate a companion. Not only that, but those who have trouble controlling their eating and weight are viewed negatively by society as having trouble controlling their basic desires.

There is this kind of psychology, but very few people will talk about it. You'll find that these problems go away when you eat properly.

Wrapping Up

There are several well-liked diets available today, but the majority of them are harmful and occasionally even dangerous. This will describe how to avoid unhealthy diets and maintain a healthy, balanced diet for life.

Find out how many calories your body needs every day to function.

Depending on your metabolism and level of physical activity, this figure may vary greatly. Your daily caloric intake should remain around 2000 calories for men and 1500 calories for women if you're the type of person who gains 10 pounds after just smelling a slice of pizza.

Additionally, your body mass affects this: For naturally bigger people, more calories are recommended, and for smaller people, fewer calories. You may want to boost your daily caloric intake by 1000–2000 calories, a little less for women, if you're the type of person who can eat without gaining weight or you're physically active.

Don't dread fatty foods.

For your body to function properly, you must consume fat from food. But it's important to choose the right kinds of fats: The majority of animal fats and a few vegetable oils are high in the LDL (bad) cholesterol-raising kind of fat.

Contrary to popular opinion, eating cholesterol doesn't always increase your body's level of cholesterol. Your body will eliminate additional cholesterol if you give it the right resources. You should strive to routinely take monounsaturated fatty acids, which are those tools. Olive oil, almonds, fish oil, and various seed oils are foods that are high in monounsaturated fatty acids.

Eat plenty of the correct curbs.

As your body relies mostly on carbohydrates for energy, you must consume foods high in carbohydrates. The problem is identifying the right crabs. The digestive tract of the body easily absorbs simple carbohydrates like sugar and refined wheat.

Your body responds by releasing massive amounts of insulin to combat the overload, which causes a kind of curb overload. In addition to harming your heart, too much insulin also promotes weight growth.

Consume a lot of crabs, but also slow-digesting foods like whole-grain flour, vegetables, oats, and unprocessed grains.

Eat bigger meals early on in the day.

As the evening wears on, your metabolism slows down and becomes less effective at breaking down meals. That means your body won't absorb as many nutrients from the meal and more of the energy included in the food will be stored as fat.

Try eating a large meal for lunch, a medium-sized meal for dinner, and a small meal for breakfast. Better still, try eating 4-6 small meals throughout the course of the day.

Provide yourself a cheat meal.

Cheating involves enjoying a food you genuinely love once a week rather than bingeing on all the wrong things once a week. On Sundays, have a few slices of pizza, and on Saturdays, eat a giant slice of double chocolate cake.

This treat meal is beneficial to your health in several ways and will help you stick to your new diet. Birthdays in the family and other special events are considered cheat meals.

Get the habit of eating slowly.

It will make you feel full with less calories while preventing overeating and obesity with all of its negative effects.

Drink plenty of H2O.

It improves your skin, awakens you and gives you more energy, and makes you feel fuller so you eat less. You will benefit greatly from reducing your soda use and switching to water.

www.ingramcontent.com/pod-product-compliance
Lightning Source LLC
LaVergne TN
LVHW052113160826
845678LV00015B/3529
* 9 7 9 8 3 7 0 0 4 3 8 1 9 *